THE HEA[...]

LEAN AND GREE[...]

FOR MEAT DISHES

50 step-by-step easy and affordable recipes for a Lean and Green food for your meat dishes to stay fit and boost energy

Josephine Reed

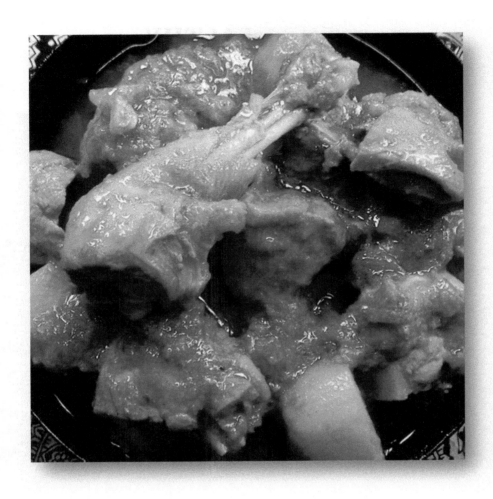

Table of contents

Orange Chicken

Prep Time: 15 minutes

Cook Time: 30 minutes

Serve: 4

Ingredients:

- 1 lb. of skinless, boneless-chicken, cut into bite-sized pieces 1/2 tsp. Crystal Light Orange Drink
- 1 tsp. of powdered garlic 1/2 tsp. Dried ground ginger 1/4 tsp. Red flakes of pepper 1/8 tsp. pepper
- 2 tsp. of olive oil
- 2 tbsp. Of rice vinegar 2 tbsp. water
- 1/2 tsp. of sesame oil
- 1 tsp. of medium soy sauce
- 1/2 tbsp. of minced dried onion 1/4–1/2 tsp. of dried orange peel

Instructions:

1.Preheat the oven to 350° C.

2.Put the chicken in a 13x9 inches baking dish.

3.In a small bowl, mix the remaining ingredients. Pour over the chicken. Bake until done, for 25–30 minutes.

Nutrition: Energy (calories): 171 kcal Protein: 25.78 g Fat: 6.06 g Carbohydrates: 1.42 g Calcium, Ca11 mg Magnesium, Mg35 mg

Salma Lime Chicken

Prep Time: 10 minutes

Cook Time: 45 minutes

Serve: 5

Ingredients:

- 5 boneless, skinless breasts of chicken 4 tbsp. of lime juice
- 1 1/4 tbsp. of chili powder 1 1/4 cup of fresh salsa

Instructions:

1.Preheat the oven to 350° C.

2.Line the foil with a 13x9 inches baking dish. Spray with non-stick cooking spray.

3.Put the chicken in your baking dish. Sprinkle the chili powder. Add lime juice and salsa.

4.Bake until done, for 40–45 minutes.

Nutrition: Energy (calories): 817 kcal Protein: 43.37 g Fat: 26.21 g Carbohydrates: 101.14 g Calcium, Ca132 mg Magnesium, Mg104 mg Phosphorus, P433 mg

Scandinavian Chicken

Prep Time: 10 minutes

Cook Time: 45 minutes

Serve: 6

Ingredients:

- 1 lb. boneless chicken breasts without skin 1 tbsp. Mrs. Dash Seasoning Original Blend 1/2 tsp. dried ground ginger
- 1/4 tsp. pepper
- 1/4 tsp. Ground cinnamon 1/4 tsp. ground nutmeg
- 1 tbsp. of olive oil
- 3 tbsp. of wine vinegar
- 1/2 tbsp. Worcestershire sauce
- 1 1/2 tbsp. Brown sugar substitute 1/2 tbsp. dried minced onion
- 1 garlic clove, hacked

Instructions:

1.Make a fire in the oven to 350° C.

2.Put the chicken in a baking dish that is 13x9 inches.

3.In a small cup, mix up the remaining ingredients. Pour the chicken over. For 45 minutes, cook.

Nutrition: Energy (calories): 169 kcal Protein: 20.71 g Fat: 7.87 g Carbohydrates: 2.11 g Calcium, Ca18 mg Magnesium, Mg18 mg

Spinach and Mushroom Stuffed Chicken

Prep Time: 20 minutes

Cook Time: 30 minutes

Serve: 4

Ingredients:

- 4 boneless skinless halves of chicken breast
- 4 softened laughing cow light cheese wedges (any flavor) 1 cup of chopped spinach
- 1 cup of white mushrooms, sliced or chopped Italian seasoning
- Parmesan cheese

Instructions:

1.Heat the oven to 350° C.

2.Fillet chicken breasts by cutting a "pocket" horizontally into the middle of the meat around ¾ of the way down, being careful not to cut through to the other side. To absorb some water within the breast, add a paper towel.

3.Place one wedge of laughing cow cheese in the middle of each breast. Cover with 1 tbsp. Of mushrooms and about 2 tbsp. Of spinach. Close them very well. If needed, secure it with a toothpick. Season with Italian seasonings (or any seasoning of your choice) and a little Parmesan cheese outside the chicken.

4.Bake for 32 minutes or until the chicken isn't pink anymore.

Nutrition: Energy (calories): 847 kcal Protein: 113.9 g Fat: 26.44 g Carbohydrates: 30.96 g Calcium, Ca252 mg Magnesium, Mg152 mg

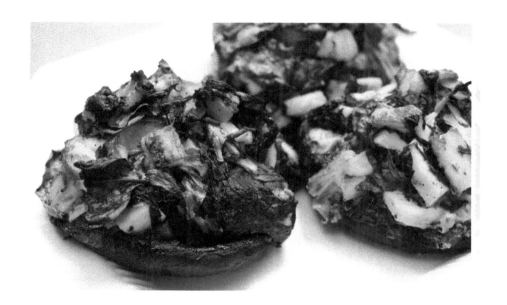

Rosemary Chicken

Prep Time: 20 minutes

Cook Time: 45 minutes

Serve: 4

Ingredients:

- 4–5 (4–6 oz.) boneless chicken breasts without skin 1/2 cup white cooking wine (or chicken broth)
- 1 tbsp. of lemon juice
- 1 1/2 tsp. Balsamic vinegar 1 tsp. Of powdered garlic 1/2 tsp. Dried rosemary 1/4 tsp. salt (optional)
- 1/8 tsp. pepper

Instructions:

1.Prepare the cooking machine to 350° C.

2.In a cookie sheet that is 13x9 inches, bring the chicken in.

3.In a small cup, mash up the best ingredients. Drop the chicken over. Cook until done, about 40-45 minutes.

Nutrition: Energy (calories): 327 kcal Protein: 47.78 g Fat: 12.92 g Carbohydrates: 2.03 g Calcium, Ca26 mg Magnesium, Mg42 mg

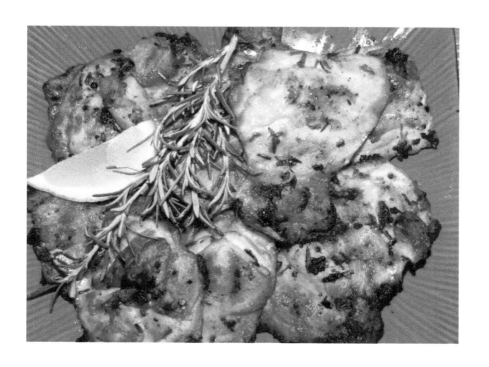

Stuffed Chicken Breasts with Tomato Salad

Prep Time: 20 minutes

Cook Time: 15 minutes

Serve: 4

Ingredients:

- 1 6.5-oz pot drained and chopped artichoke hearts 2 tbsp. grated parmesan
- 2 spoonsful of new thyme leaves
- 4 6-oz boneless, skinless breasts of chicken 2 tbsp. + 1 tsp. extra-virgin olive oil Pepper and kosher salt
- 2 beefsteak tomatoes, sliced into bite-sized bits 1 shallot, sliced thinly
- 1 tablespoon red wine vinegar
- 8 toasted baguette slices (optional)

Instructions:

1.In a small cup, combine the artichokes, parmesan, and 1 tablespoon of thyme.

2.Cut a 2-inch pocket into each chicken breast's thickest section. Use a quarter of the artichoke mixture to stuff each bag.

3.With 1 teaspoon of oil, rub the chicken breasts and season with a three-fourth teaspoon of salt and one-fourth teaspoon of pepper.

4.Heat the grill or barbecue pan to medium. Grill the chicken for 7 minutes, turning once, until cooked through.In a wide bowl, mix the tomatoes, shallot, vinegar, one-fourth teaspoon of salt and pepper, and the remaining oil and thyme.

5.If needed, slice the chicken and, if desired, serve with the tomato salad and baguette slices.

Nutrition: Energy (calories): 1818 kcal Protein: 63.07 g Fat: 134.17 g Carbohydrates: 114.55 g Calcium, Ca425 mg Magnesium, Mg960 mg Phosphorus, P2234 mg

Super-fast Chicken Salad Sandwich

Prep Time: 20 minutes

Cook Time: 0 minutes

Serve: 2

Ingredients:

- 2 cans of chicken (3 oz. each), rinsed and drained twice 1 celery stick, finely chopped
- 1 tbsp. Onion, finely chopped 1 tbsp. of pine nuts
- 1 tsp. of spicy brown mustard
- 1 heaping tsp. of sour cream free of fat 1 heaping tsp. of plain yogurt free of fat Ground black pepper pinch
- 4 whole-grain bread slices 2 lettuce leaves

Instructions:

1.Combine the celery, onion, pine nuts, vinegar, sour cream, yogurt, and pepper in a dish. Mix the chicken in.

2.On a slice of bread, spread out half of the mixture. Place a lettuce leaf on top and then another slice of bread on top.

3.To make a second sandwich, repeat with the remainder of the mixture.

Nutrition: Energy (calories): 764 kcal Protein: 34.8 g Fat: 50.96 g Carbohydrates: 40.18 g Calcium, Ca131 mg Magnesium, Mg94 mg

Quick and Easy Protein Salad

Prep Time: 20 minutes

Cook Time: 0 minutes

Serve: 2

Ingredients:

- 2 cups of baby spring mix 2 chopped scallions
- ½ cucumber, cut in half and sliced 4 spores, halved and cut
- 1/4 of a medium avocado, diced
- 1/2 cup of cottage cheese free of fat 1 hardboiled egg, diced
- 1 lemon juice
- 1 garlic clove, minced
- 3 tbsp. low-fat buttermilk
- Salt and ground black pepper, to taste

Instructions:

1.In a medium-sized mixing bowl, add the spring mix, scallions, cucumber, mushrooms, avocado, cottage cheese, hardboiled egg, and toss. Switch to a wide tray.

2.In a little-mixing bowl, add the lemon juice, garlic, buttermilk, salt, pepper, and incorporate well.

3.Work over the salad with the sauce.

Nutrition: Energy (calories): 628 kcal Protein: 60.98 g Fat: 27.46 g Carbohydrates: 33.82 g Calcium, Ca355 mg Magnesium, Mg102 mg

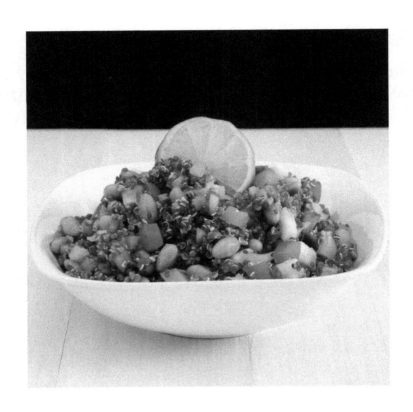

Feta Chicken with Zucchini

Prep Time: 20 minutes

Cook Time: 20 minutes

Serve: 2

Ingredients:

- 2 tbsp. olive oil 1 lemon
- 4 boneless, skinless-chicken breasts (about 1 1/2 lb.) One-fourth tsp. kosher salt
- 2 mid-sized zucchinis
- One-fourth cup fresh, chopped flat-leaf parsley leaves 13 tsp. of black pepper
- One-third cup of crumbled Feta (about 2 oz.)

Instructions:

1.Heat the furnace to 400° F. In a roasting pan, drizzle one-half tablespoon of the oil. In thin stripes, remove the skin from the lemon; set aside. Slice the lemon thinly. In the pan, place half the slices.

2.On top of the lemon slices, place the chicken and season with 1/8 of a teaspoon of salt.

3.Lengthwise, split each zucchini in half, then split each half into one-fourth inch-thick half-moons. Combine the zucchini, parsley, pepper, the remaining oil, slices of lemon, salt in a bowl; toss.

4.Spread the mixture over the chicken and sprinkle it over the top with the Feta.

5.Roast for 16 to 21 minutes until the chicken is fully cooked. Switch it to a cutting board and cut it into thirds for each piece.

6.Divide the chicken, zucchini mixture, and lemons between individual plates, and sprinkle with the zest.

Nutrition: Energy (calories): 2176 kcal Protein: 111.16 g Fat: 88.45 g Carbohydrates: 236.31 g Calcium, Ca819 mg Magnesium, Mg343 mg

Cinnamon Chicken

Prep Time: 20 minutes

Cook Time: 20 minutes

Serve: 2

Ingredients:

- 4 or 5 (4-6 oz.) boneless chicken breasts without skin 2 tbsp. Italian Dressing Low-Calorie
- 1 tsp. of cinnamon
- 1 1/2 tsp. Powdered garlic 1/4 tsp. salt (optional)
- 1/4 tsp. pepper

Instructions:

1.Heat the oven the 350 ° C oven.

2.In a 13x9 baking dish, bring the chicken in. Pour the Italian sauce over it.

3.Blend the remaining ingredients in a small bowl. Sprinkle chicken over it. Bake for 40–45 minutes.

Nutrition: Protein: 94.9 g Fat: 26.29 g Carbohydrates: 6.69 g Calcium, Ca66 mg Magnesium, Mg79 mg Phosphorus, P552 mg

Chinese Five Spice Chicken

Prep Time: 20 minutes

Cook Time: 20 minutes

Serve: 2

Ingredients:

- 2 entire chicken breasts bone-in, with skin 2 tsp. of five-spice Chinese powder
- 1 tsp. Of powdered garlic, Salt and pepper, for taste 1 tbsp. olive oil

Instructions:

1.Rinse the breasts and pat the chicken dry. Sprinkle with garlic powder, five-spice powder, salt, and pepper. Cover securely in aluminum foil and cool for at least 2 hours to marinate.

2.Bring to fire your oven to 175° C (350° F).

3.Remove the wrapping from the chicken breasts and put them in a 9x13 inches baking dish that is lightly greased.

4.Drizzle with olive oil and bake for 46 minutes at 350° F (175° C), or until the juices are cooked through and clear.

Nutrition: Energy (calories): 572 kcal Protein: 61.02 g Fat: 33.68 g Carbohydrates: 3.01 g Calcium, Ca45 mg Magnesium, Mg81 mg

Chicken with Acorn Squash and Tomatoes

Prep Time: 20 minutes

Cook Time: 20 minutes

Serve: 2

Ingredients:

- 1 little-acorn squash (about 1 1/2 lb.), 1/4 inch thick, halved, seeded, and sliced
- 1 pint of grape tomatoes, halved 4 garlic cloves, cut
- 3 tbsp. olive oil
- Black pepper and kosher salt
- 4 6-oz boneless, skinless breasts of chicken One-half tsp. ground cilantro
- 2 tbsp. of fresh oregano, chopped

Instructions:

1.Heat the furnace to 425° F.

2.Toss the squash, tomatoes, and garlic with 2 little spoons of oil, one-half teaspoon of salt, and one-fourth teaspoon of pepper on a broad-rimmed baking sheet.

3.Roast the vegetables for 21 to 25 minutes until the squash is tender.

4.Meanwhile, over medium heat, heat the remaining tablespoon of oil in a large skillet.

5.Season the coriander, one-half teaspoon salt, and one-fourth teaspoon pepper with the poultry. Cook, 6 to 7 minutes per hand, until golden brown and cooked through.

6.Serve the squash and tomatoes with the chicken and sprinkle with the oregano.

Nutrition: Energy (calories): 877 kcal Protein: 34.11 g Fat: 39.9 g Carbohydrates: 98.08 g Calcium, Ca165 mg Magnesium, Mg144 mg

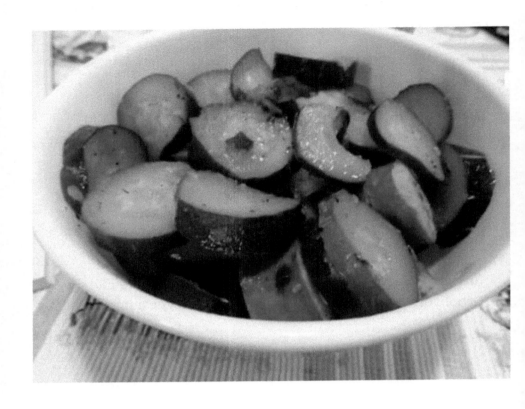

Chicken Cordon Blue

Prep Time: 15 minutes

Cook Time: 20 minutes

Serve: 2

Ingredients:

- 2 4-oz boneless chicken breasts, skinless,
- 2 large leaves of spinach, washed, stems removed 2 wedges laughing cow light cheese
- 1 oz. of reduced-ham without nitrate sodium Paprika, to taste
- 1 garlic clove, minced
- 1 tsp. of extra-virgin olive oil
- 1 cup Baby Bella mushrooms, sliced 1/8 tsp. ground black pepper
- 2 tsp. yogurt sauce
- 1/2 cup Greek nonfat yogurt 1 tbsp. Dijon mustard
- 1/2 tsp. buttermilk
- 2 tbsp. chives, chopped

Instructions:

1.Set up the oven to 400° F.

2.Pound the chicken with a mallet till it is 1/4-inch thick. Take care not to rip a breast apart.

3.On top of each breast lay 1 spinach leaf. Spread a slice of cheese to cover the spinach. Top with 1/2 slice of ham and fold the ham over to match the breast as desired.

4.Roll each breast up gently and protect it with a toothpick. Sprinkle with paprika on the outer side of the breast. Bake for 20 minutes in the oven until the chicken is completely cooked.

5. Sauté the garlic in the oil in a non-adhesive skillet over medium-high heat for 1 minute while the chicken is cooking. Add pepper and mushrooms. Stir regularly until soft for 10 minutes. Withdraw from the sun. Cover and set aside.

6.Whisk together the yogurt, mustard, and buttermilk for sauce preparation. Mix the chives in.

7.Divide the mushrooms evenly, about 1/4 cup each, between 2 plates. Then put the chicken on the mushroom bed and drizzle the top with 1/4 cup of yogurt sauce.

Nutrition: Energy (calories): 180 kcal Protein: 29.41 g Fat: 5.35 g Carbohydrates: 1.95 g Calcium, Ca21 mg Magnesium, Mg42 mg

Chicken Kampala

Prep Time: 15 minutes

Cook Time: 1 and 1/2 hours

Serve: 4-5

Ingredients:

- 3 lbs. chicken parts
- 2 tbsp. butter
- 2 tbsp. olive oil
- 2 med. Onions, chopped two cloves garlic, minced 1 c. canned tomatoes
- 3 oz. tomato paste
- 2 sticks cinnamon
- 1/4 tsp. Ground allspice 1/4 tsp. sugar
- 1/4 c. red wine

Instructions:

1.Heat 2 tbsp. Butter, and 1 tbsp. Olive-oil in a skillet and add the chicken—Cook chicken over medium heat for about 15 minutes, often stirring to keep chicken from burning. Take it out of the skillet once the chicken is browned and apply the remaining butter and oil to the pan.

2.Ensure the skillet is still hot before adding the onions and cooking for about 5 minutes over medium heat. Stir in the garlic and tomatoes, cooking for another 5 minutes. Stir in the tomato paste, cinnamon, allspice, sugar, red wine, and chicken, including juices.

3.Bring to a boil and cover tightly (you can use foil and cover with foil). Reduce heat and simmer, occasionally stirring, for 1 and 1/2 hours.

4.Serve with white rice.

Nutrition: Energy (calories): 421 kcal Protein: 56.41 g Fat: 17.51 g Carbohydrates: 6.43 g Calcium, Ca46 mg Magnesium, Mg73 mg

Garlic and Citrus Turkey with Mixed Greens

Prep Time: 5 minutes

Cook Time: 15 minutes

Serve: 4

Ingredients:

- 4 teaspoons (or oil of your choice and fresh chopped garlic) 1 C scallion greens, thinly sliced
- 1 3/4 pounds lean ground turkey
- 1 Tablespoon (or lemon, pepper, garlic, onion, parsley, salt & pepper)
- 8 cups mixed green lettuce
- 1 lemon cut into wedges for garnish

Instructions:

1.Heat a large non-stick skillet with oil and sauté the garlic over medium-high heat for 1 minute, stirring.Add scallion greens, green onions, ground turkey, and seasonings. Stir and cook for 16 minutes, or until meat is thoroughly cooked.

2.Divide greens between 4 plates and top each plate with 1/4 of the meat mixture.

3.Serve with lemon wedges.

Nutrition: Energy (calories): 355 kcal Protein: 38.71 g Fat: 21.33 g
Carbohydrates: 3.54 g Calcium, Ca81 mg Magnesium, Mg57 mg
Phosphorus, P421 mg

Greek Chicken with Yogurt

Prep Time: 10 minutes

Cook Time: 20 minutes

Serve: 4

Ingredients:

- oil spray
- 5 oz. plain Greek yogurt 2 tbsp mayonnaise
- 1/2 cup grated parmesan-cheese 1 tsp garlic powder
- 1/4 tsp salt
- 1/4 tsp black-pepper
- 1.5 lb. chicken-tenders (whole) or chicken-breasts (cut in quarters) Parsley (chopped, for garnish)

Instructions:

1. Fire up the oven to 480 degrees F.

2. Line a baking sheet with parchment paper. Spray oil on parchment, then place chicken on top (the oil will help prevent the chicken from sticking to the parchment paper).

3. In a little-mixing bowl, whisk together the yogurt, mayo, parmesan, garlic powder, salt, and pepper. Toss the chicken

tenders or breasts with the yogurt mixture and place them on the baking sheet.

4.Repeat with the remaining chicken and yogurt/spices mixture.

5.For 20 minutes, bake. Garnish with extra parsley and immediately serve sprinkled on top with extra Greek yogurt, mayo, and grated parmesan.

Nutrition: Energy (calories): 325 kcal Protein: 42.78 g Fat: 14.13 g Carbohydrates: 4.87 g Calcium, Ca189 mg Magnesium, Mg60 mg

Sliced Steak with Canadian Crust

Prep Time: 10 minutes

Cook Time: 20 minutes

Serve: 5

Ingredients:

- 10-ounce steaks good for grilling (ask your butcher for suggestions) about 1 and one-half thick
- 1 Tablespoon (1 Capful) (or other dry steak seasonings)

Instructions:

1.Preheat broiler

2.Sprinkle on both sides of steak dry steak seasonings seasoning

3.Place steak under pre-heated broiler

4.Broil each side to taste (approx. 5 minutes per side for medium-rare)

5.Slice steak in thin, 3/4" slices against the grain.

6.Arrange slices on a serving platter and top with a generous amount of butter.

Nutrition: Energy (calories): 51 kcal Protein: 6.58 g Fat: 2.02 g Carbohydrates: 1.03 g Calcium, Ca7 mg Magnesium, Mg8 mg

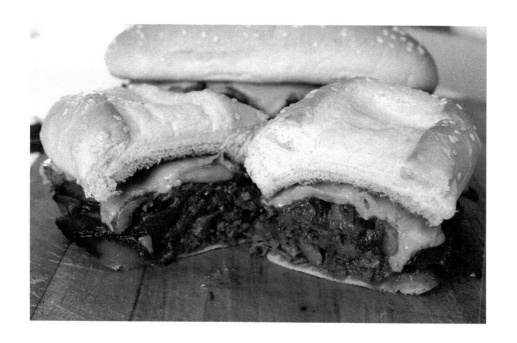

BBQ Chicken with Sesame Ginger "Rice"

Prep Time: 10 min and refrigerate for 3 h up to overnight.

Cook Time: 12 minutes

Serve: 4

Ingredients:

- 4 (4 to 6 ounces each) boneless (skinless-chicken breasts) For the Marinade:
- 1/2 cup soy-sauce
- 3 garlic cloves (peeled and crushed) 1/4 cup seasoned rice wine vinegar 2 normal spoons honey
- 1 normal spoon fresh ginger root (peeled and grated) 4 medium green onions (chopped)
- 2 normal spoons toasted sesame oil 1 little spoon toasted sesame seeds
- Garnish: 2 normal spoons whole fresh cilantro leaves

Instructions:

1.Using a mallet, pound the chicken until 1/2 inch thick. Cut into 1-inch strips.

Preparation:

2.Place the chicken in a resealable bag.

3.In a 9x13x2 baking pan, mix the soy sauce, garlic, Rice Vinegar, honey, and ginger. Add the chicken-breasts and turn to coat. Seal with a non-reactive covering. Refrigerate for 3 hours up to overnight.

4.Preheat a gas grill to medium-high heat. Discard the marinade and remove the chicken

5.Arrange the chicken strips on the grill pan with tongs to cook for 8 to 12 minutes until the chicken is thoroughly cooked. DO NOT overcook. The chicken is done when the juices-run clear. Transfer the chicken to a platter. Cover with foil and set aside (if finishing later).

6.In a medium casserole dish, add the ¼ cup water and bring to a boil. Stir in the sesame oil, sesame seeds, and the rice vinegar and salt.

7.While the rice is cooking, prepare the barbecue-cooked chicken.

8.To serve, divide the chicken strips among 4 servings.

Nutrition: Energy (calories): 268 kcal Protein: 8.75 g Fat: 13.55 g Carbohydrates: 28.93 g Calcium, Ca43 mg Magnesium, Mg39 mg Cholesterol14 mg

Fork Tender Beef Goulash with Peppercorn & Sage

Prep Time: 15 minutes

Cook Time: 35 minutes

Serve: 4

Ingredients:

- 2 Tbsp Olive oil
- 2 Onions, chopped roughly 4 garlic cloves, crushed
- 2 Celery stalks, sliced
- 800 g Beef rump steaks, or use stewing steak, cut into 3cm cubes 1 Tbsp Paprika
- ½ bottle Red wine
- 1 tin Chopped tomato, approx. 420g 1 Tbsp Balsamic vinegar
- 1/2 Peppercorn
- 2 tsp Brown sugar
- 1 stalk Sage, leaves only 1 pinch Chili flakes
- 1 pottle Sour cream, for serving

Instructions:

46

1.In a heavy saucepan, sauté the onion, celery, and garlic till soft. Add the meat and brown well.

2.Set aside a small amount of the meat, sliced thinly, and return the rest to the pan along with the paprika, wine, chopped tomatoes, balsamic vinegar, and sugar.

3.Preheat the oven to 160°C.

4.Gently simmer for 20–30 minutes, adding the whole peppercorn and sage bundle. With a sharp knife, remove the peppercorn and sage.

5.Increase the heat and simmer vigorously for another 10 minutes.

6.Serve garnished with the reserved meat slices, sour cream, and chili flakes.

Nutrition: Energy (calories): 417 kcal Protein: 44.36 g Fat: 18.21 g Carbohydrates: 17.78 g Calcium, Ca58 mg Magnesium, Mg73 mg Phosphorus, P507 mg

Simple Sonoma Skillet

Prep Time: 15 minutes

Cook Time: 30 minutes

Serve: 4

Ingredients:

- 4 teaspoons of your choice of oil
- 1 cup scallions (or onions if permitted in your program) 1 cup red-bell-pepper, thinly sliced
- 1 cup of yellow-bell pepper, thinly sliced
- Thinly cut 20 ounces-chicken or steak (can be cooked leftovers or uncooked)
- Stacey Hawkins Phoenix Sunrise Seasoning 1 normal-spoon (one capful)

Instructions:

1.Put a big-skillet on medium heat and let it heat up.

2.Add the extra virgin olive oil and the scallion or onion, and thinly sliced bell peppers.

3.Sauté them for about 5 minutes until they start to soften.

4.Add the meat and let it cook for 6 minutes or so until it's no longer pink.

5.Add the Phoenix Sunrise Seasoning.

6.Cook for a few more minutes, and it is ready to serve.

Nutrition: Energy (calories): 307 kcal Protein: 38.65 g Fat: 12.37 g Carbohydrates: 8.49 g Calcium, Ca43 mg Magnesium, Mg42 mg Phosphorus, P360 mg

Italian Chicken with White Wine, Peppers, and Anchovy

Prep Time: 10 minutes

Cook Time: 25 minutes

Serve: 4

Ingredients:

FOR THE CHICKEN

- 1 normal spoon olive oil
- 4 boneless-skinless chicken breasts salt and fresh ground pepper to taste 1 little spoon garlic powder
- 1 tablespoon anchovy

FOR THE SMOOTH SAUCE OF WHITE WINE

- 1 regular spoon of unsalted butter 1 diced large-yellow onion 3 minced garlic cloves
- Salt and fresh ground pepper, 1 cup of dry white wine to taste
- 1 dried thyme small-spoon
- New chopped parsley
- 1/2 cup half-and-half/heavy cream/evaporated milk

Instructions:

1.Pan Heat the olive oil in a heavy large skillet over medium-high heat. Season the chicken with salt, pepper garlic powder and combine it with the anchovy flakes. Ad the chicken to the pan and cook on both sides until it is golden brown. Ensure that you are sauteing in the pan, lower the heat to keep from burning.

2.Magnetic Mixer Dispersion Whip the wine, thyme, garlic, pepper, and salt in a glass bowl. Add the cream, mix in the cubes of butter. Keep mixing for a few minutes, and then add the peppers. Keep mixing and cook the fusion.

3.Mixer-ext. Ended Hand Cut the chicken into strips (or very small pieces if desired. The pieces are easier to eat). Combine the chicken with the mixture—Cook the fusion for 10 minutes. Serve with pasta or on warm pieces of French bread.

Nutrition: Energy (calories): 742 kcal Protein: 110.07 g Fat: 26.87 g Carbohydrates: 9.25 g Calcium, Ca262 mg Magnesium, Mg150 mg Phosphorus, P1171 mg

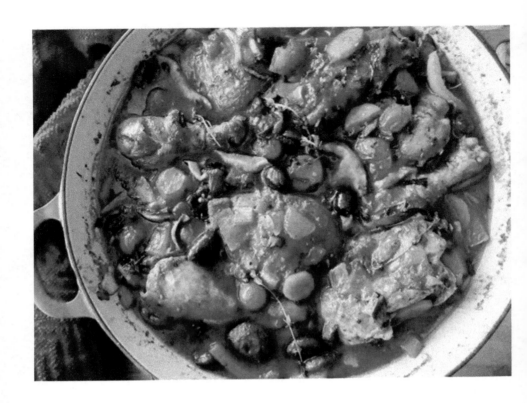

Tagine of Chicken and Olives

Prep Time: 10 minutes and marinate for 3-4 hours

Cook Time: 45 minutes

Serve: 4

Ingredients:

- 5 cloves garlic, finely chopped
- One-fourth teaspoon saffron threads, pulverized One-half teaspoon ground ginger
- 1 teaspoon sweet paprika
- Half a little-spoon of ground cumin, half a teaspoon of turmeric
- 1 chicken, salt and freshly ground black pepper, cut into 8 to 10 pieces.
- 3 medium onions, sliced thin, 2 tablespoons extra virgin olive oil
- 1 cinnamon stick
- 8 pitted and halved kalamata olives
- 8 cracked green, pitted and halved olives
- 1 big or 3 small lemons preserved (sold in specialty food shops) 1 cup of stock of chicken

- 1/2 lemon juice
- 1 tablespoon of flat-leaf parsley chopped

Instructions:

1.In a big-plastic food bag, combine the garlic, saffron, ginger, parsley, paprika, cumin, turmeric, salt, and pepper. To coat the spices with the chicken, add the chicken and shake the bag. Set it aside for 1 hour to 3 hours to marinate.

2.Transfer the chicken to a large pot and add the remaining ingredients. If there isn't any liquid in the bag, add enough water to cover the pot's ingredients. Cover and cook for 36 to 46 minutes, until the chicken is tender and the liquid is reduced.3.Serve garnished with lemon juice and parsley.

Nutrition: Energy (calories): 1090 kcal Protein: 115.01 g Fat: 64.59 g Carbohydrates: 6.08 g Calcium, Ca111 mg Magnesium, Mg137 mg

Citrus Chicken

Prep Time: 10 minutes

Cook Time: 3-4 hour

Serve: 3

Ingredients:

- 6 bone-in chicken breast halves, 1 tea separated from the flesh.
- 1/2 teas seasoned salt 1/4 teas pepper
- 2 Tbsp olive oil 1/4 cup water
- 3 Tbsp lemon juice
- 2 garlic cloves, minced
- 1 teas chicken bouillon granule 2 teas minced fresh parsley

Instructions:

1.Rinse chicken; pat dry. Place chicken in a 4-qt. Slow cooker.

2.Combine the oregano, seasoned salt, pepper, oil, water, lemon juice, garlic, bouillon, and parsley; pour over the chicken.

3. Cover and cook until tender, for 3-4 hours or until the chicken is tender.

Nutrition: Energy (calories): 1379 kcal Protein: 151.74 g Fat: 80.84 g Carbohydrates: 1.75 g Calcium, Ca86 mg Magnesium, Mg140 mg

Chunky Chicken Pie

Prep Time: 10 minutes

Cook Time: 30 minutes

Serve: 3

Ingredients:

- 3 boneless skinless chicken breasts 2 tablespoons sunflower oil
- 300 ml of milk
- 200 ml chicken stock (it's okay from a cube) 2 tablespoons of flour
- Fifty g of butter
- 1 clove of garlic, hacked
- 1 tablespoon of chopped freshly grated nutmeg parsley
- About salt
- 1 Shortcrust pastry ready to roll, rolled eggs moderately thinly pounded, glazed

Instructions:

1. Pounding with a rolling pin on the chicken breasts with until they are about three to eight thick and set aside. Cook the garlic in the oil in a saucepan until it is pale yellow.

2.Precisely Mix the flour and everything, add to the oil and cook for 5 minutes over low heat, stirring at first, until the flour turns clear and the dish is thick. Add the nutmeg and season with salt, mix well. Take the pan from the heat and let it cool slightly. Add this to the chicken breasts to obtain a heavy pin.

3.Shape into a square by covering them with wax paper and pounding them with a rolling pin. Spread the chicken mixture evenly over the pastry. Roll the pastry's edges over the outsides of the chicken mixture to form a rim and bake in a preheated hot oven 220 ° C. until golden brown, about 20 minutes. Serve hot with fresh vegetables.

Nutrition: Energy (calories): 10597 kcal Protein: 614.33 g Fat: 511.1 g Carbohydrates: 867.92 g Calcium, Ca14044 mg Magnesium, Mg1576 mg

Tender Rosemary Pork Chops

Prep Time: 15 minutes

Cook Time: 20 minutes

Serve: 4   .

Ingredients:

- 4 pork loin chops kosher salt
- Freshly ground black pepper
- 1 tbsp. freshly minced rosemary 2 cloves garlic, minced
- 1/2 c. (1 stick) butter melted 1 tbsp. extra-virgin olive oil

Instructions:

1.Preheat grill or broiler with 1/2 inch of oil in the pan.

2.With paper towels, pat the chops dry, and season with salt and pepper to taste.

3.Brush the chops with the melted butter and sprinkle the rosemary and garlic over them on both sides.

4.Grill the chops for 20 minutes or until tenderness comes

5.Serve with a simple carrot and red bell pepper medley.

Nutrition: Energy (calories): 547 kcal Protein: 40.57 g Fat: 41.81 g
Carbohydrates: 0.6 g Calcium, Ca49 mg Magnesium, Mg41 mg
Phosphorus, P355 mg

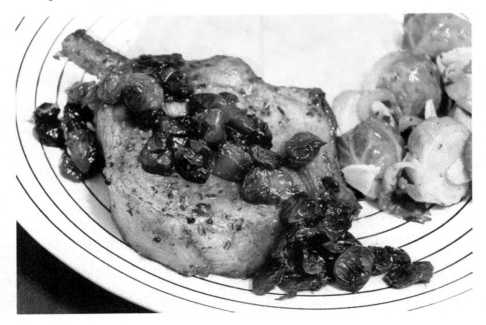

Tomatillo and Green Chili Pork Stew

Prep Time: 15 minutes

Cook Time: 30 minutes

Serve: 1

Ingredients:

- 1/2 scallions, chopped
- 1/2 cloves of garlic
- 1/4 pound tomatillos, trimmed and chopped
- 2 large romaine or green lettuce leaves, divided
- 1/2 serrano chilies, seeds, and membranes
- ½ teaspoon dried Mexican oregano (or you can use regular oregano)
- 1/4 pound of boneless pork loin, to be cut into bite-sized cubes
- ¼ cup coriander, chopped
- ¼ tablespoon (each) salt and paper
- 1/4 jalapeno, seeds, and membranes to be removed and thinly sliced
- 1/4 cup sliced radishes
- 1 lime wedge

Instructions:

1. Combine scallions, garlic, tomatillos, four lettuce leaves, serrano chilies, and oregano in a blender. Then puree until smooth.

2. Put pork and tomatillo mixture in a medium pot. 1-inch of puree should cover the pork; if not, add water until it covers it. Season with pepper & salt, and cover it simmers. For 20 minutes, let it simmer on low heat.

3. Now, finely shred the remaining lettuce leaves.

4. When the stew is done cooking, garnish with coriander, radishes, finely shredded lettuce, sliced jalapenos, and lime wedges.

Nutrition: Calories: 370, Protein: 36g, Carbohydrates: 14g, Fats: 19g

Cloud Bread

Prep Time: 30 minutes

Cook Time: 30 minutes

Serve: 1

Ingredients:

- 1/4 cup fat-free 0%
- Plain Greek yogurt (4.4 oz)
- 1 egg, separated
- 1/32 teaspoon cream of tartar
- 1/2 packet sweetener (a granulated sweetener just like stevia)

Instructions:

1. For about 30 minutes before making this meal, place the Kitchen Aid Bowl and the freezer's whisk attachment.

2. Preheat your oven to 30 degrees.

3. Eliminate the bowl and whisk attachment from the freezer.

4. Separate the eggs. Now put the egg whites in the Kitchen Aid Bowl, and they should be in a different medium-sized bowl.

5. In the medium-sized bowl containing the yolks, mix in the sweetener and yogurt.

6. In the bowl containing the egg white, add in the cream of tartar. Beat this mixture until the egg whites turn to stiff peaks.

7. Now, take the egg yolk mixture and carefully fold it into the egg whites. Be cautious and avoid over-stirring.

8. On a parchment paper, place it on a baking tray and spray with cooking spray.

9. Scoop out six equally sized "blobs" of the "dough" onto the parchment paper.

10. Bake for about 25–35 minutes (make sure you check when it is 25 minutes, in some ovens, they are done at this timestamp). You will know they are done as they will get brownish at the top and have some crack.

11. Most people like them cold against being warm.

12. Most people like to re-heat in a toast oven or toaster to get them a little bit crispy.

Nutrition: Calories: 0, Protein: 0g, Carbohydrates: 0g, Fats: 0g

Rosemary Cauliflower Rolls

Prep Time: 15 minutes

Cook Time: 30 minutes

Serve: 1 (3 biscuits per serving)

Ingredients:

- 1/12 cup almond flour
- 1 cup grated cauliflower
- 1/12 cup reduced-fat, shredded mozzarella or cheddar cheese
- 1/2 eggs
- 1/2 tablespoons fresh rosemary, finely chopped
- ½ teaspoon salt

Instructions:

1. Preheat your oven to 4000F.

2. Into a medium-sized dish, pour all the ingredients.

3. Scoop cauliflower mixture into 12 evenly sized rolls/biscuits onto a lightly greased and foil-lined baking sheet.

4. Bake until it turns golden brown, which should be achieved in about 30 minutes.

5. Note: if you want to have the outside of the rolls/biscuits crisp, then broil for some minutes before serving.

Nutrition: Calories: 138, Protein: 11g, Carbohydrates: 8g, Fats: 7g

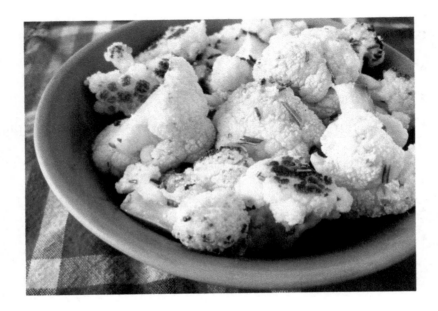

Tomato Braised Cauliflower with Chicken

Prep Time: 15 minutes

Cook Time: 30 minutes

Serve: 1

Ingredients:

- 1 garlic clove, sliced
- 3/4 scallions, to be trimmed and cut into 1-inch pieces 1/8 teaspoon dried oregano
- 1/8 teaspoon red pepper flakes
- 1/4 cups cauliflower
- 3/4 cups diced canned tomatoes
- 1/4 cup fresh basil, gently torn
- 1/8 teaspoon each of pepper and salt, divided
- 3/4 teaspoon olive oil
- 3/4 pound boneless, skinless chicken breasts

Instructions:

1. Get a saucepan and combine the garlic, scallions, oregano, crushed red pepper, cauliflower, tomato, and add ¼ cup of water. Get everything boil together, add ¼ teaspoon of pepper and salt

for seasoning, and then cover the pot with a lid. Let it simmer for 10 minutes and stir as often as possible until you observe that the cauliflower is tender. Now, wrap up the seasoning with the remaining ¼ teaspoon of pepper and salt.

2. Using olive oil, toss the chicken breast and let it roast in the oven with the heat of 4500F for 20 minutes and an internal temperature of 1650F. Allow the chicken to rest for like 10 minutes.

3. Now slice the chicken and serve on a bed of tomato-braised cauliflower.

Nutrition: Calories: 290, Fats: 10g, Carbohydrates: 13g, Protein: 38g

Cheeseburger Soup

Prep Time: 15 minutes

Cook Time: 30 minutes

Serve: 1

Ingredients:

- 1/16 cup chopped onion
- 1 quantity of (14.5 oz) can dice a tomato
- ¼ pound 90% lean ground beef
- 3/16 cup chopped celery
- 1/4 teaspoons Worcestershire sauce
- 1/2 cup chicken broth
- 1/8 teaspoon salt
- 1/4 teaspoon dried parsley
- 2/3 cups of baby spinach
- 1/8 teaspoon ground pepper
- 1 oz. reduced-fat shredded cheddar cheese

Instructions:

1. Get a large soup pot and cook the beef until it becomes brown. Add the celery, onion, and sauté until it becomes tender. Make sure to drain the excess liquid.

2. Stir in the broth, tomatoes, parsley, Worcestershire sauce, pepper, and salt. Cover and wait for it to simmer on low heat for about 20 minutes.

3. Add spinach and leave it to cook until it becomes wilted in about 1–3 minutes. Top each of your servings with 1 oz of cheese.

Nutrition: Calories: 400, Carbohydrates: 11g, Protein: 44g, Fats: 20g

Braised Collard Beans in Peanut Sauce with Pork Tenderloin

Prep Time: 25 minutes

Cook Time: 35 minutes

Serve: 1

Ingredients:

- 1/2 cups chicken stock
- 3 cups chopped collard greens
- 1 1/2 tablespoons powdered peanut butter
- 3/4 cloves of garlic, crushed
- 1/4 teaspoon salt
- 1/8 teaspoon allspice
- 1/8 teaspoon black pepper
- 1/2 teaspoons lemon juice
- 3/8 teaspoon hot sauce
- 1/8 pound pork tenderloin

Instructions:

1. Get a pot with a tight-fitting lid and combine the collards with the garlic, chicken stock, hot sauce, and half of the pepper and salt. Cook on low heat for about 1 hour or until the collards become tender.

2. Once the collards are tender, stir in the allspice, lemon juice. And they have powdered peanut butter. Keep warm.

3. Season the pork tenderloin with the remaining pepper and salt, and broil in a toaster oven for 10 minutes when you have an internal temperature of 1450F. Make sure to turn the tenderloin every 2 minutes to achieve an even browning all over. After that, you can take away the pork from the oven and allow it to rest for like 5 minutes.

4. Slice the pork as you will like and serve it on top of the braised greens.

Nutrition: Calories: 320, Fats: 10g, Carbohydrates: 15g, Protein: 45g

Zucchini Pizza Casserole

Prep Time: 15 minutes

Cook Time: 50–60 minutes

Serve: 1

Ingredients:

- ¼ teaspoon salt
- ¼ cup grated parmesan cheese
- 1/2 eggs
- 2/3 cups shredded unpeeled zucchini (this is about two medium zucchinis)
- 1 oz. reduced-fat, shredded cheddar cheese, divided
- 1 oz. reduced-fat, shredded mozzarella cheese, divided 1/8 pound 90–94% of lean ground beef
- Cooking spray
- 1 quantity 14.5 oz. can petite diced Italian tomatoes
- 1/8 cup chopped onion
- 1/2 small green bell pepper, chopped

Instructions:

1. Preheat your oven to over 4000F.

2. Place zucchini in a strainer and sprinkle it with salt. Let it stand for about 10 minutes, and after that, press it to drain its moisture.

3. Combine zucchini with eggs, parmesan, and half of cheddar cheese and mozzarella.

4.In a lightly greased baking dish, press the mixture and bake for about 20 minutes when uncovered.

5. Cook the onion and beef in a medium skillet until it becomes done. Drain any leftover liquid, and then stir in the tomatoes.

6. Pour the beef mixture over the zucchini and sprinkle with the remaining mozzarella cheese and cheddar. Top with green pepper

7. Bake for an extra 20 minutes or until it becomes heated all through.

Nutrition: Calories: 478, Protein: 30g, Carbohydrates: 22g, Fats: 29g

Tofu Power Bowl

Prep Time: 10 minutes

Cook Time: 15–20 minutes

Serve: 1

Ingredients:

- 15 oz. extra-firm tofu
- 1 teaspoon rice vinegar
- 2 tablespoons soy sauce
- 1 teaspoon sesame oil
- ½ cup grated cauliflower
- ½ cup grated eggplant
- ½ cup chopped kale

Instructions:

1. Press tofu. Place tofu strips in multiple layers of paper towel or a clean dishcloth on top of a cutting board or plate. On top of the tofu, put another clean dish towel or paper towel. Place a weight on top of this second layer (this can be a large plate with canned foods on top or hardcover books, or a stack of leaves). Let it sit for not less than 16 minutes, and then cut the tofu into 1-inch cubes.

2. Combine both the vinegar and soy sauce in a small bowl and whisk together.

3. Get a large skillet and heat the sesame oil in it. Place cubed tofu to cover one half of the skillet, and the cubed eggplant should cover the other half. Cook both together until they become slightly brown and tender in about 10–12 minutes. Remove from skillet and keep aside. Now, add kale and sauté until they become wilted in about 3–5 minutes.

4. Microwave the already grated cauliflower in a small bowl with one teaspoon of water for about 3–4 minutes until it becomes tender.

5. Arrange the cauliflower "rice" with tofu, eggplant, and kale in a bowl.

Nutrition: Calories: 117, Protein: 14g, Carbohydrates: 2.2g, Fats: 7g

Grilled Veggie Kabobs

Prep Time: 15 mi

Cook Time: 12 to 15 min

Serve: 1

Ingredients:

Marinade:

- ½ cup balsamic vinegar
- 1/3 tablespoons minced thyme
- 1/4 tablespoons minced rosemary
- 1/2 cloves garlic, peeled and minced
- Sea salt, to taste (optional)
- Freshly ground black pepper, to taste

Veggies:

- 1/3 cups cherry tomatoes
- 1/3 red bell pepper, it should be seeded and cut into 1-inch pieces 1/3 green bell pepper, without seeds and cut into 1-inch pieces 1/3 medium yellow squash, cut into 1-inch rounds
- 1/3 medium zucchini, cut into 1-inch rounds
- 1/3 medium red onion skinned and cut into large chunks

Special Equipment:

- Two bamboo skewers, make sure to soak it in water for 30 minutes.

Instructions:

1. Preheat the grill to medium heat.

2. In making the marinade: In a small bowl, stir together the balsamic vinegar, thyme, rosemary, garlic, salt (if desired), and pepper.

3. Thread veggies onto skewers, alternating between different-colored veggies.

4. Grill the veggies for 12 to 15 minutes until softened, and lightly it was charred, brushing the veggies with the marinade and flipping the skewers every 4 to 5 minutes.

5. Remove from the grill and serve hot.

Nutrition: Calories: 98, Fat: 0.7g, Carbs: 19.2g, Protein: 3.8g, Fiber: 3.4g

Grilled Cauliflower Steaks

Prep Time: 10 minutes

Cook Time: 57 minutes

Serve: 1

Ingredients:

- 1/2 medium heads cauliflower
- 1/2 medium shallots, peeled and minced Water, as needed
- 1/2 clove garlic, peeled and minced
- ½ teaspoon ground fennel
- ½ teaspoon minced sage
- ½ teaspoon crushed red pepper flakes
- ½ cup green lentils, rinsed
- 1/2 cups low-sodium vegetable broth
- Salt, to taste (optional)
- Freshly ground black pepper, to taste
- Chopped parsley, for garnish

Instructions:

1. On a flat work surface, cut each of the cauliflower heads in half through the stem, then trim each half, so you get a 1-inch-thick steak.

2. Arrange each piece on a baking sheet and set aside. You can reserve the extra cauliflower florets for other uses.

3. Sauté the shallots in a medium saucepan over medium heat for 10 minutes, stirring occasionally. Add water, 1 to 3 tablespoons at a time, to keep the shallots from sticking.

4. Stir in the garlic, fennel, sage, red pepper flakes, and lentils and cook for 3 minutes.

5. Pour into the vegetable broth and bring to a boil over high heat.

6. Reduce the heat to medium, cover, and cook for 45 to 50 minutes, or until the lentils are very soft, adding more water as needed.

7. Using an immersion blender, purée the mixture until smooth. Sprinkle with salt (if desired) and pepper. Keep warm and set aside.

8. Preheat the grill to medium heat.

9. Grill the cauliflower steaks for about 7 minutes per side until evenly browned.

10. Transfer the cauliflower steaks to a plate and spoon the purée over them. Serve garnished with the parsley.

Nutrition: Calories: 105, Fat: 1.1g, Carbs: 18.3g, Protein: 5.4g, Fiber: 4.9g

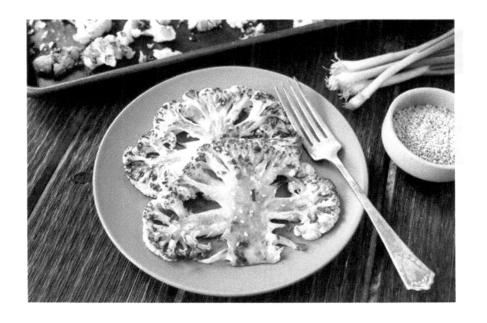

Vegetable Hash with White Beans

Prep Time: 15 minutes

Cook Time: 23 minutes

Serve: 1

Ingredients:

- 1 leek (white part only), finely chopped
- 1 red bell pepper, deseeded and diced
- Water, as needed
- 2 teaspoons minced rosemary
- 3 cloves garlic, peeled and minced
- 1 medium sweet potato, peeled and diced
- 1 enormous turnip, peeled and diced
- 2 cups cooked white beans
- Zest and juice of 1 orange
- 1 cup chopped kale
- Salt, to taste (optional)
- Freshly ground black pepper, to taste

Instructions:

1. Put the leek and red pepper in a large saucepan over medium heat and sauté for 8 minutes, stirring occasionally. Add water, 1 to

3 tablespoons at a time, to keep them from sticking to the bottom of the pan.

2. Stir in the rosemary and garlic and sauté for 1 minute more.

3. Add the sweet potato, turnip, beans, and orange juice and zest, and stir okay—heat until the vegetables are softened.

4. Add the kale and sprinkle with salt (if desired) and pepper. Cook for about 5 minutes or more until the kale is wilted.

Nutrition: Calories: 245, Fat: 0.6g, Carbs: 48.0g, Protein: 11.9g, Fiber: 9.3g

Salad Mix

Prep Time: 20 minutes

Cook Time: 25 minutes

Serve: 1

Ingredients:

- 1 medium red onion, peeled and diced
- Water, as needed
- 4 cloves garlic, peeled and minced
- 1 medium red bell pepper, without seeds and diced
- 1 small zucchini, diced
- 1 medium eggplant stemmed and diced
- 1 large tomato, diced
- ½ cup chopped basil
- Salt, to taste (optional)
- Freshly ground black pepper, to taste

Instructions:

1. Put the onion in a medium saucepan over medium heat and sauté for 10 minutes, stirring occasionally, or until the onion is tender. Add water 1 to 3 tablespoons at a time to keep it from sticking.

2. Add the garlic, red pepper, zucchini, and eggplant and stir well. Lid the saucepan and cook for 12 to 15 minutes, stirring occasionally.

3. Mix in the tomatoes and basil, then sprinkle with salt (if desired) and pepper. Serve immediately.

Nutrition: Calories: 76, Fat: 0.5g, Carbs: 15.3g, Protein: 2.7g, Fiber: 5.9g

Indian Spiced Eggplant

Prep Time: 15 minutes

Cook Time: 25 minutes

Serve: 1

Ingredients:

- 1/2 medium onions, peeled and diced
- 1/4 medium red bell pepper, deseeded and diced Water, as needed
- 1/2 large tomatoes, finely chopped
- 1/2 medium eggplants, stemmed, peeled, and cut into ½-inch dices
- 3/4 tablespoons grated ginger
- 1/4 teaspoon coriander seed, toasted and ground
- 1/2 teaspoons cumin seeds, toasted and ground
- ½ teaspoon crushed red pepper flakes
- Pinch cloves
- Salt, to taste (optional)
- 1/2 coriander, leaves, and tender stems, finely sliced

Instructions:

1. Combine the onions and red pepper in a large saucepan and cook over medium heat for about 10 to 12 minutes. Include water 1 to 2 tablespoons now to keep them from sticking to the pan.

2. Stir in the tomatoes, eggplant, ginger, coriander, cumin, crushed red pepper flakes, and cloves and cook for just about 12 to 15 minutes, or until the vegetables are tender.

3. Sprinkle with the salt, if desired. Garnish with the coriander.

Nutrition: Calories: 140, Fat: 1.1g, Carbs: 27.9g, Protein: 4.7g, Fiber: 10.9g

Kale and Pinto Bean Enchilada Casserole

Prep Time: 10 minutes

Cook Time: 30 minutes

Serve: 1

Ingredients:

- 1/2 teaspoon olive oil (optional)
- 1/2 yellow onion, diced
- 1/2 bunch kale stemmed and chopped
- 1/4 teaspoons taco seasoning
- 1/2 to 2/3 cups cooked pinto beans, or 2 (15-oz./425-g) cans pinto beans, drained and rinsed
- Sea salt, to taste (optional)
- Black pepper, to taste
- 1/2 (16-oz./454-g) jar salsa (any variety), divided
- 2 corn tortillas
- ½ cup cashew cheese, or more to taste

Instructions:

1. Preheat the oven to 350ºF (205ºC). Grease a baking dish with the olive oil, if desired.

2. Place the onion, kale, taco seasoning, and beans in the dish. Then sprinkle with salt (if desired) and pepper. Drizzle half the salsa over the beans. Next, place the tortillas on top. Scatter with the remaining salsa and cashew cheese.

3. Before baking, cover the dish with aluminum foil in the preheated oven for about 30 minutes or until the vegetables are warm and the salsa bubbles.

4. Let it cool for 10 minutes before slicing and serving.

Nutrition: Calories: 194, Fat: 3.8g, Carbs: 29.0g, Protein: 10.9g, Fiber: 9.4g

Potato and Zucchini Casserole

Prep Time: 10 minutes

Cook Time: 1 hour

Serve: 1

Ingredients:

- 1/2 large russet potatoes halved lengthwise and thinly sliced
- 1/2 medium zucchinis halved lengthwise and thinly sliced 1/4 cup nutritional yeast
- 1/4 cup diced green or red-bell-pepper (about one small bell pepper)
- 1/4 cup diced red, white, or yellow onion (about one small onion) 1/8 cup dry breadcrumbs
- 1/8 cup olive oil (optional)
- 2/3 teaspoons minced garlic (about three small cloves)
- Pepper, to taste
- Sea salt, to taste (optional)

Instructions:

1. Preheat the oven to 400ºF.

2. Mix all the ingredients.

3. Place the mixture in a large cooking pot dish.

4.Bake in the preheated oven for 55 minutes until heated through, stirring once halfway through.

5. Remove and allow to cool from the oven before serving for 5 minutes.

Nutrition: Calories: 352, Fat: 10.0g, Carbs: 51.5g, Protein: 14.1g, Fiber: 5.5g

Broccoli Casserole with Beans and Walnuts

Prep Time: 10 minutes

Cook Time: 35–40 minutes

Serve: 1

Ingredients:

- 1/4 cup vegetable broth
- 1/2 broccoli heads, crowns, and stalks finely chopped 1/3 teaspoon salt (optional)
- 2/5 cups cooked pinto or navy beans
- 1/2 to 2/3 tablespoons brown rice flour or arrowroot flour
- 1/4 cup chopped walnuts

Instructions:

1. Preheat the oven to 410ºF (205ºC).

2. Warm the vegetable broth in a large ovenproof pot over medium heat.

3. Add the broccoli and season with salt, if desired, then cook for 6 to 8 minutes, stirring occasionally, or until the broccoli is light green.

4. Add the pinto beans and brown rice flour to the skillet and stir well. Sauté for another 5 to 7 minutes, or until the liquid thickens slightly. Scatter the top with the walnuts.

5. Transfer the pot to the oven. Bake it until the walnuts are toasted, 20 to 25 minutes.

6. Let the casserole cool for 8 to 10 minutes in the pot before serving.

Nutrition: Calories: 412, Fat: 20.2g, Carbs: 43.3g, Protein: 21.6g, Fiber: 13.1g

Pistachio Crusted Tofu

Prep Time: 10 minutes

Cook Time: 20 minutes

Serve: 1

Ingredients:

- 1/8 cup roasted, shelled pistachios
- 1/8 cup whole-wheat breadcrumbs
- 1/4 garlic clove, minced
- 1/4 shallot, minced
- 1/8 teaspoon dried tarragon
- 1/4 teaspoon grated lemon zest
- Sea salt, to taste (optional)
- Black pepper, to taste
- 1/4 (16-oz./454-g) package sprouted or extra-firm tofu, drained and sliced lengthwise into eight pieces
- 1/8 tablespoon dijon mustard
- 1/8 tablespoon lemon juice

Instructions:

1. Warm up the oven to 400ºF (205ºC). Line a baking sheet with parchment paper.

2. Then, place the pistachios in a food processor until they are about the breadcrumbs' size. Mix the pistachios, breadcrumbs, garlic, shallot, tarragon, and lemon zest in a shallow dish. Sprinkle with salt (if desired) and pepper. Set aside.

3. Sprinkle the tofu with salt (if desired) and pepper. Mix the mustard and lemon juice in a small bowl and stir well.

4. Brush all over the tofu with the mustard mixture, then coat each slice with the pistachio mixture.

5. Arrange the tofu on the baking sheet. Scatter any remaining pistachio mixture over the slices.

6. Bake in the warmed oven for about 18 to 20 minutes, or until the tofu is browned and crispy.

Nutrition: Calories: 159, Fat: 9.3g, Carbs: 8.3g, Protein: 10.4g, Fiber: 1.6g

Air Fryer Asparagus

Prep Time: 5 minutes

Cook Time: 8 minutes

Serve: 1

Ingredients:

- Nutritional yeast
- Olive oil non-stick spray
- 1 bunch of asparagus

Instructions:

1. Prepare the ingredients. Wash asparagus. Do not forget to trim off thick, woody ends.

2. Spray asparagus with olive oil spray and sprinkle with yeast.

3. Air Frying. In your Instant Crisp Air Fryer, lay asparagus in a singular layer. Set the temperature to 360°F. While the time limit to 8 minutes.

Nutrition: Calories: 17, Fat: 4g, Protein: 9g

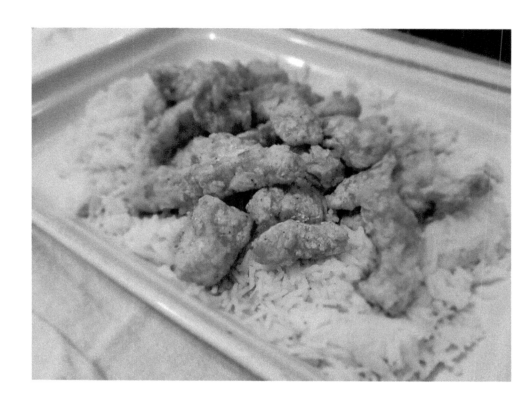

Avocado Fries

Prep Time: 10 minutes

Cook Time: 7 minutes

Serve: 1

Ingredients:

- 1 avocado
- 1/8 teaspoon salt
- 1/4 cup panko breadcrumbs
- Bean liquid (Aquafaba) from a 15- oz. can of white or garbanzo beans

Instructions:

1. Prepare the ingredients. Peel, pit, and slice up avocado.

2. In a tub, toss the salt and breadcrumbs together. Put the aquafaba in a separate tub.

3. First in Aquafaba and then in panko, dredge slices of avocado, ensuring you can also cover them.

4. Air Frying. Place coated avocado slices into a single layer in the Instant Crisp Air Fryer. Set temperature to 390°F and set time to 5 minutes.

5. Serve with your favorite Keto dipping sauce!

Nutrition: Calories: 102, Fat: 22g, Protein: 9g, Sugar: 1g

Cauliflower Rice

Prep Time: 5 minutes

Cook Time: 20 minutes

Serve: 1

Ingredients:

Round 1:

- 1/2 teaspoon turmeric
- 1/2 cup diced carrot
- 1/8 cup diced onion
- 1/2 tablespoon low-sodium soy sauce
- 1/8 block extra firm tofu

Round 2:

- ½ cup frozen peas
- 1/4 minced garlic cloves
- ½ cup chopped broccoli
- 1/2 tablespoon minced ginger
- 1/4 tablespoon rice vinegar
- 1/4 teaspoon toasted sesame oil
- 1/2 spoon reduced-sodium soy sauce 1/2 cup riced cauliflower

Instructions:

1. Prepare the ingredients. Crush tofu in a large bowl and toss with all the round one ingredient.

2. Air Frying. Lock the air fryer lid. Preheat the Instant Crisp Air Fryer to 370 degrees. Also, set the temperature to 370°F, set the time to 10 minutes, and cook 10 minutes, making sure to shake once.

3. In another bowl, toss ingredients from round 2 together.

4. Add round 2 mixture to Instant Crisp Air Fryer and cook another 10 minutes to shake 5 minutes.

Nutrition: Calories: 67, Fat: 8g, Protein: 3g, Sugar: 0g

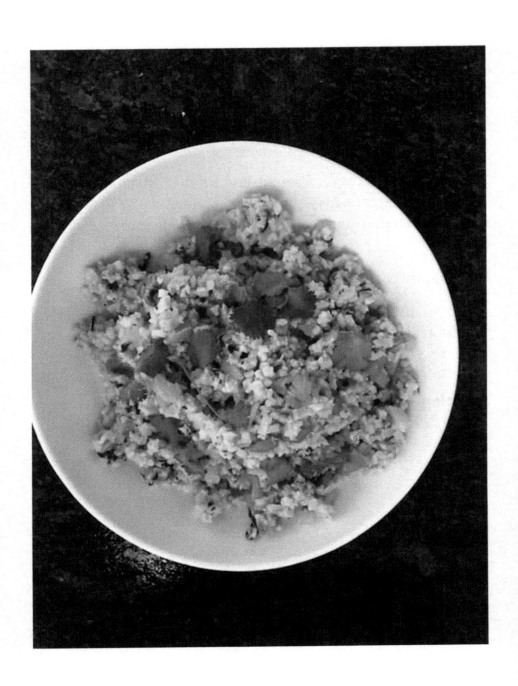

Stuffed Mushrooms

Prep Time: 7 minutes

Cook Time: 8 minutes

Serve: 1

Ingredients:

- 1/2 rashers bacon, diced
- ½ onion, diced
- ½ bell pepper, diced
- 1/2 small carrot, diced
- 2 medium-size mushrooms (Separate the caps & stalks)
- 1/4 cup shredded cheddar plus extra for the top 1/4 cup sour cream

Instructions:

1. Prepare the ingredients. Chop the mushrooms stalks finely and fry them up with the bacon, onion, pepper, and carrot at 350F° for 8 minutes.

2. Also, check when the veggies are tender, stir in the sour cream & the cheese. Keep on the heat until the cheese has melted and everything is mixed nicely.

3. Now grab the mushroom caps and heap a plop of filling on each one.

4. Place in the fryer basket and top with a little extra cheese.

Nutrition: Calories: 285, Fat: 20.5g, Protein: 8.6g

Zucchini Omelet

Prep Time: 10 minutes

Cook Time: 10 minutes

Serve: 1

Ingredients:

- 1/2 teaspoon butter
- 1/2 zucchini, julienned
- 1 egg
- 1/8 teaspoon fresh basil, chopped
- 1/8 teaspoon red pepper flakes, crushed Salted and newly ground black pepper, to taste

Instructions:

1. Prepare the ingredients. Preheat the Instant Crisp Air Fryer to 355ºF.

2. Melt butter on medium heat using a skillet.

3. Add zucchini and cook for about 3–4 minutes.

4. In a bowl, add the eggs, basil, red pepper flakes, salt, and black pepper and beat well.

5. Add cooked zucchini and gently stir to combine.

6. Air Frying. Transfer the mixture into the Instant Crisp Air Fryer pan. Lock the air fryer lid.

7. Cook for about 10 minutes. Also, you may opt to wait until it is done thoroughly.

Nutrition: Calories: 285, Fat: 20.5g, Protein: 8.6g

Cheesy Cauliflower Fritters

Prep Time: 10 minutes

Cook Time: 7 minutes

Serve: 1

Ingredients:

- ½ cup chopped parsley
- 1 cup Italian breadcrumbs
- 1/3 cup shredded mozzarella cheese
- 1/3 cup shredded sharp cheddar cheese
- 1 egg
- 2 minced garlic cloves
- 3 chopped scallions
- 1 head of cauliflower

Instructions:

1. Prepare the ingredients. Cut the cauliflower up into florets. Wash well and pat dry. Place into a food processor and pulse 20–30 seconds until it looks like rice.

2. Place the cauliflower rice in a bowl and mix with pepper, salt, egg, cheeses, breadcrumbs, garlic, and scallions.

3. With hands, form 15 patties of the mixture, then add more breadcrumbs if needed.

4. Air Frying. With olive oil, spritz patties, and put the fitters into your Instant Crisp Air Fryer. Pile it in a single layer. Lock the air fryer lid. Set temperature to 390°F, and set time to 7 minutes, flipping after 7 minutes.

Nutrition: Calories: 209, Fat: 17g, Protein: 6g, Sugar: 0.5

Zucchini Parmesan Chips

Prep Time: 10 minutes

Cook Time: 8 minutes

Serve: 1

Ingredients:

- ½ teaspoon paprika
- ½ cup grated parmesan cheese
- ½ cup Italian breadcrumbs
- 1 lightly beaten egg
- 2 thinly sliced zucchinis

Instructions:

1. Prepare the ingredients. Use a very sharp knife or mandolin slicer to slice zucchini as thinly as you can. Pat off extra moisture.

2. Beat egg with a pinch of pepper and salt and a bit of water.

3. Combine paprika, cheese, and breadcrumbs in a bowl.

4. Dip slices of zucchini into the egg mixture and then into the breadcrumb mixture. Press gently to coat.

5. Air Frying. With olive oil cooking spray, mist encrusted zucchini slices. Put into your Instant Crisp Air Fryer in a single layer. Latch the air fryer lid. Set temperature to 350°F and set time to 8 minutes.

6. Sprinkle with salt and serve with salsa.

Nutrition: Calories: 211, Fat: 16g, Protein: 8g, Sugar: 0g

Crispy Roasted Broccoli

Prep Time: 10 minutes

Cook Time: 8 minutes

Serve: 1

Ingredients:

- ¼ teaspoon masala
- ½ teaspoon red chili powder
- ½ teaspoon salt
- ¼ teaspoon turmeric powder
- 1 tablespoon chickpea flour
- 1 tablespoon yogurt
- ½ pound broccoli

Instructions:

1. Prepare the ingredients. Cut broccoli up into florets. Immerse in a bowl of water with two teaspoons of salt for at least half an hour to remove impurities.

2. Take out broccoli florets from water and let drain. Wipe down thoroughly.

3. Mix all other ingredients to create a marinade.

4. Toss broccoli florets in the marinade. Cover and chill for 15–30 minutes.

5. Air Frying. Preheat the Instant Crisp Air Fryer to 390 degrees. Place marinated broccoli florets into the fryer, lock the air fryer lid, set the temperature to 350°F, and set the time to 10 minutes. Florets will be crispy when done.

Nutrition: Calories: 96, Fat: 1.3g, Protein: 7g, Sugar: 4.5g

Lightning Source UK Ltd.
Milton Keynes UK
UKHW020706130521
383649UK00005B/58